The Fabu Naturals Fat Burner Diet

Burn Fat & Lose Weight While

Eating What You Want in 3 Easy Steps

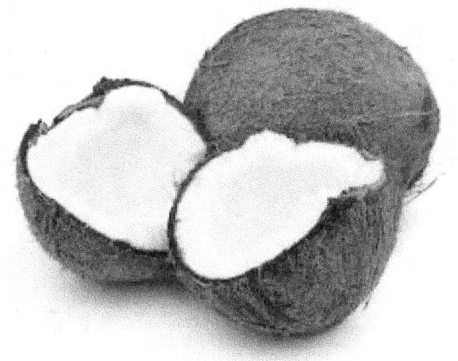
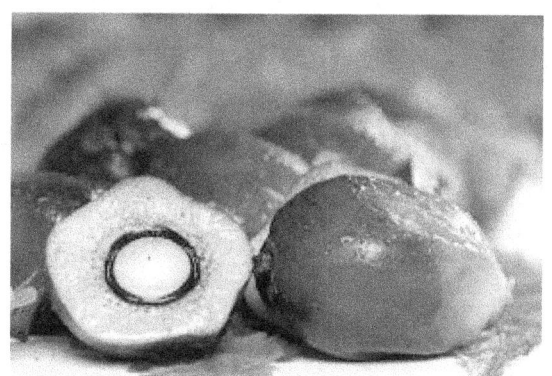

Bernique M. Johnson

Founder & CEO of Fabu Naturals

Table Of Contents

Introduction

For months I tried every diet pill and plan on the market without success. As I have Fibromyalgia it is impossible for me to do strenuous exercise which has been a big impediment to losing weight because you have to move to burn fat. Also due to Fibroids, soy products were completely out of the question for use in my diet. As a vegetarian, getting my daily allowance of protein, which is a fat burner in itself, was also a challenge. But I finally found a way to lose 30 pounds in 3 months in 3 easy steps.

I stumbled on coconut/palm oil in an article from Dr. Oz. It comes in many different forms from water to milk to flour to sugar to flakes for baking. Coconut, in all it's forms, is a source of fiber, vitamins, minerals, amino acids, calcium, potassium and magnesium.

The oil keeps skin looking young and beautiful and can help to slow the aging processes by protecting your skin against free radicals and can help to treat skin conditions like eczema, psoriases and dermatitis.

It helps keep hair strong and shiny, helps maintain strong bones and teeth due to its high calcium and magnesium content and is an alternative for lactose intolerant individuals.

Coconut and palm oils come from the palm tree family. Coconut oil is temperature sensitive, meaning it's solid in cold temperatures and liquid in warm temperatures. Palm oil is non-hydrogenated and is always solid until it's melted. Once it's melted it will never become solid again. Coconut oil is also more expensive than Palm oil.

Both are saturated fats but unlike animal fats, coconut & palm oils are not deposited in the body as fat globules. They are sent immediately to the liver and burned for energy increasing your metabolism thus making them excellent oils for weight loss as they are only burning the fat already in your body instead of contributing to more of it.

Once I discovered the fat burning and weight loss potential of coconut/palm oil, I set out to create a diet program that I felt would help me lose the weight I needed to lose.

Introduction

After additional research I discovered Pacific Oat Milk (shameless unpaid plug) which is made from the same oats you eat in oatmeal and contains 10 vitamins, 15 minerals, iron, more calcium and vitamin A than cows milk, contains only on 2.5g of fat with no saturated fat, and is lactose & cholesterol free which makes it an excellent alternative for lactose intolerant individuals.

It's also is a remedy for the nervous system which helps keep you calm, is diabetic friendly and can be made from scratch if necessary.

I also discovered Greek yogurt made with a combination of cow's milk and goat's milk. The difference between Greek yogurt and regular yogurt is that the whey (the watery milky substance left after the milk is curdled and strained) is strained from Greek yogurt and is kept in regular yogurt.

Greek yogurt contains 50% less sodium, is low in carbohydrate (9g vs. 15-17g in regular yogurt) is easily digestible and good for lactose intolerant people, due to its low level of lactose and sugar, live cultures and probiotic (beneficial micro organisms) properties, is delicious to people who don't like yogurt (like myself) and can be substituted for sour cream in baking.

Goat's milk can be fattening in large amounts but also will increase your metabolism. It's high in calcium, B2 or Riboflavin, which is key to gaining and maintaining energy, contains anti-inflammatory compounds and protein molecules smaller than the molecules in cow's milk which, makes it easier to digest for people allergic to cow's milk including infants and children.

Simple Truth Greek Yogurt (a Kroger brand) (shameless unpaid plug) is the only brand I know that combines the two and the yogurt and flavoring are separate which is great for diabetics. Greek yogurt is higher in protein than regular yogurt which helps you feel full.

If Simple Truth or a brand similar to it is not available in your local grocery or health food store you can make you own by combining 1 part goat's milk Greek yogurt to 3 parts cow's milk Greek yogurt.

Introduction

Additional research directed me to flax, a blue flowered herbaceous plant cultivated for it's seeds which are loaded with nutritional benefits and fiber. Just 2 tablespoons delivers 4 grams of fiber, as much as 1 ½ cups of cooked oatmeal. It lowers LDL and maintains a healthy level of HDL cholesterol.

Flax seed contains 75% more lignans than other seeds, which are chemical compounds found in plants, and are classified as a major phytoestrogen which means it mimics estrogen when broken down by the digestive system. It also acts as an anti-oxidant.

Flax contains omega 3 fatty acids and is heart healthy. The benefits can only be obtained from ground flax seeds, oil or milk. Use flax seed sparingly as it's a powerful laxative and can cause diarrhea if used in large quantities.

Finally I discovered Coconut Water which is a great high potassium hydrator & diuretic from the young green coconut. It's electrolyte composition is almost identical to human plasma and was used as such during World War II. It's a great hydrator, so great that I have to remember to drink water during the day as I'm never really thirsty

I combined these ingredients to make a protein shake that I used as the foundation of my weight loss plan.

The ingredients seem to combine to work synergistically to increase the metabolism, burn fat, remove water weight and help to fill you up so you are not as hungry during the day which makes it easier to stay on the diet.

On the following pages I will outline in detail the protein shake, diet and exercise plan I used to lose 30 pounds in 3 months.

Create Your Diet Plan

Before you start you first need to determine your daily caloric intake. The amount of calories you need to eat everyday in order to lose weight. The best way to determine that is to use one of the many online calorie counters. I recommend Livestrong.com/myplate (another shameless unpaid plug) as it not only determines your caloric intake it also helps you to design your meal & exercise program to gain the maximum benefits of this diet.

Once you have determined how much weight you want to lose and how fast you want to lose it, you get on with the plan.

Notes for Success.

I am a vegetarian but I will add diet modifications for non-vegetarians.

Coconut oil has about 110 calories and palm oil has about 120 calories per tablespoon. But Don't Panic. Since they are delivered directly to the liver instead of your body they won't contribute to weight gain when consumed in moderation.

This is a high protein, low carbohydrate diet. So when planning your meals make sure you are eating as much protein and as few carbohydrate as possible by the end of each day. Being vegetarian takes extra work to meet even your minimum daily protein requirement let alone go above it, so be sure to take advantage of all the non-meat protein alternatives that are available from both your grocery and health food stores. Drinking milk with dinner will help to add protein and help to fill you up. As a reference our Facebook page contains articles & listings of many protein alternatives.

About Plateauing. Once your body gets used to a certain calorie level you will stop losing weight. It happened to me throughout my experience. While it's frustrating I was able to overcome it and jumpstart my weight loss again by adding no more than 200 extra calories over my daily caloric intake for 2 days. Normally I would do it on 1 weekend by eating breakfast along with my shake. The weight loss would resume during the week. This is only to jumpstart your metabolism and weight loss again, not every weekend.

Always talk to your doctor before starting any diet plan.

The Diet Plan

Step 1

The most important part of the diet is the exercise program. You have to move to lose weight. I lost my weight just by walking 90 minutes a day, 7 days a week. Online calorie counters like Livestrong.com/myplate calculates calories burned from different levels of exercise so be sure to include calories burned from your exercise regiment when you are planning your caloric intake for the day. With the extra calories I burned from walking, I was able to increase my daily caloric intake so as to ensure that I did not feel deprived.

Step 2

The second most important part of the diet is to replace your animal and/or vegetable oils with coconut or palm oil every day. In other words no butter, margarine, animal or vegetable shortening or oils. You will cook, fry and bake with either coconut oil or palm oil. You can also substitute coconut flour (dried, ground, powdered coconut meat) & coconut sugar (the sap from coconut blossoms reduced to crystal form with heat) for regular flour and sugar in baked goods, frosting and glaze recipes. Coconut flour and sugar can be found in your local grocery or health food store. As coconut flour does not contain gluten, it cannot be a one for one substitute for flour. Replace up to 20% of unbleached flour with coconut flour depending on the recipe. As coconut flour is drier and more fibrous than flour you will also have to add an extra equal amount of liquid. A blender or food processor can grind granulated sugar into powdered sugar.

I found that coconut oil is best for baking as it makes your baked goods extra moist and oiling your pan or dish with palm oil will ensure that your baked goods won't stick to the pan & dishwashing will be a breeze. Palm oil works best for cooking, frying and flaky pie crusts because of it's high heat tolerance while imparting a non-stick benefit to your cooking. Palm or coconut oil can eliminate the need for silicone based cooking sprays for all of your cooking and baking needs. Spectrum (another shameless unpaid plug) is an excellent choice for both coconut & palm oil and can be found both in your local grocery or local health food store.

The Diet Plan

Step 3

The third most important part of the diet is to drink the protein shake once a day and eat what you like. Just make sure you don't exceed your calories for the day. The Livestrong.com/myplate contains a database of most prepackaged and fresh foods and gives you the complete nutritional value of each food type to plan your meals and calorie intake for the day This way you can either cook from scratch, dine out, or eat the prepackaged foods you love to eat while just replacing the oil with coconut or palm. Just decide what you are going to eat each day whether it's home cooked, restaurant or prepackaged and enter it into the Livestrong database. It will automatically calculate calories for the day.

Note:

Prepackaged foods contain large amounts of salt, sugar, animal and vegetable oils & preservatives, which is something you must take into account when planning your meals for your diet. I recommend cooking from scratch whenever possible so you can control your salt, sugar & fat intake and it's healthier.

When eating meat choose chicken, turkey or fish primarily. When eating red meat choose cuts that are as lean as possible and prepare them in either coconut or palm oil. You will lose weight faster when you are not adding a lot of extra fat that must be burned and lost.

Drink plenty of water. This diet contains herbs and foods that have diuretic properties and a lack of adequate water can cause bloating.

Finally! The Protein Shake

This shake contains around 300 calories which must be factored into your daily caloric intake but remember the calories from the coconut milk & water are not turned into fat globules but is burned in the liver as energy to increase your metabolism.

1/3 cup Oat Milk

1/3 cup Coconut Water

1/3 cup Coconut Milk

1 container Simple Truth Greek Yogurt in your favorite flavor (You can substitute 1 part Greek goat's milk yogurt to 3 parts cows milk Greek yogurt) or you can use your favorite Greek yogurt. (As I only used Simple Truth I don't know if using other brands of yogurt will affect the calorie burning aspect of the shake.)

Pinch of Flax Seed Meal

1 Tablespoon granulated sugar (or a sweetener of your choice, which is optional, but recommended if you are using goat's milk yogurt as goat's milk is not as sweet as cow's milk)

Add oat milk, coconut water, coconut milk & yogurt (without flavoring) into a blender.

Set on stir and add sweetener, flax seed meal & flavoring while blender is stirring. When using separate fruits with yogurt keeping the blender on prevents the fruit flavoring from settling in the bottom of the blender. You can also add fresh fruit to your shake if you want. Finally place blender on whip until the fruit/flavoring is completely incorporated into the shake. Pour into a glass and enjoy.

Only drink 1 shake per day. You can drink it any time of day but I recommend it as breakfast since it does help with hunger pains. Do not eat breakfast with the shake. You can drink coffee or tea.

Finally! The Protein Shake

Should you need to snack during the day the 100 calorie snacks at stores are available along with rice cakes, fruit and/or vegetables. Remember these will count towards your daily calorie intake so you should add it to your meal plan. Chickweed tea is also an excellent appetite suppressant & healthy diuretic and can be found at your local health food store. Also drinking plenty of water will help to fill you up while helping to flush toxins out of your body.

Everyone's metabolism is different but following the diet plan of 1 shake per day along with exercise and a good meal plan within my daily caloric intake I initially lost 8 pounds in the 1st 7 days. After that I lost approximately 1 to 2 pounds a week. Your results may be more or less dramatic but the goal is to continue to lose your weight steadily until you reach your weight goal.

Become Successful On This Diet

The ingredients in the protein smoothie have been proven to provide great weight loss results. In case you chose to use other types of milk or oat milk is not available in your area, I've listed other alternatives you may use. You can also find recipes for making your own oat milk online. I cannot vouch for the smoothie's effectiveness using these other milk alternatives.

Milk Alternatives

Rice Milk

Rice milk is a lactose free and non-allergenic milk alternative that is low fat, loaded with vitamins and mineral such as vitamin B-6, Iron, Copper and Magnesium. It can be used for cooking. The downside is its low protein, high carbohydrate & low calcium.

Almond Milk

Almond milk is a nutty flavored milk alternative that can be used for cooking and drinking. It contains as much calcium and vitamin D as dairy milk. It's rich in potassium, manganese, magnesium, vitamin E, copper & selenium. It's low in saturated fat with no cholesterol and is low calorie.

Cashew Milk

Is high in B vitamins (thiamin, riboflavin, niacin & B6), copper, magnesium, heart healthy, low fat and cholesterol free.

Nut milks should not be used by individuals with nut allergies.

Sunflower Milk

Sunflower milk is made from the seeds and contains high levels of vitamin E, strong antioxidant and anti-inflammatory properties, vitamins B1, B5, magnesium, calcium, zinc, manganese, copper, selenium, phosphorous, omega 3 amino acids and phytosterols. It's helps lower cholesterol and boosts cardiovascular health.

Become Successful On This Diet

Margarine Substitutes

Earth Balance Buttery Spread

The best margarine substitute I've used is (another shameless unpaid plug) Earth Balance Natural Buttery Spread. There are several options and they taste like butter, have zero trans fat, is vegan, non-GMO, gluten free, non-dairy and can be used just like butter or margarine in all your favorite foods.

Butter Buds/Cheese Sprinkles

Butter Buds are an all natural dehydrated butter powder with 10 calories and zero fat. It's great for zero calorie popcorn, eggs, potatoes, any food where you add margarine or butter.

Cheese Sprinkles are made from dehydrated cheese in powder form also with low calories which tastes like cheese and is great low calorie alternative for popcorn, spaghetti and other foods.

Sweeteners

These are the six major sugar alternatives

Stevia

Stevia comes from a plant and can be used just like sugar in cooking, seasoning and baking. It's low calorie, low glycemic (good for diabetics) and good for people with high blood pressure. It has an after taste but many millions of people use Stevia for all their sweetening needs.

Maple Syrup

Maple Syrup can (surprisingly) be used as a sugar substitute in cooking and baking and contains many health benefits such as promoting heart health and boosting the immune system.

Become Successful On This Diet

Honey

You can't go wrong with honey. It's a naturally low glycemic sweetener that's rich in antioxidants and can treat insomnia, beautify the skin, help heal wounds and promotes good digestion.

Agave Nectar

Agave nectar is extracted from the same agave plant and nectar used to make Tequila. Available in light and dark, this (in my opinion) is the closest and best sugar alternative. It tastes sweeter than sugar, is low glycemic and can contribute to weight loss, relieve inflammation, boost the immune system and improve absorption of calcium, magnesium and isoflavones.

Date Sugar

Date sugar is not really sugar at all but the dehydrated extract taken from dates. It's a healthy sugar substitute and contains iron, calcium, phosphorous, magnesium, zinc, and selenium. It helps maintain blood pressure, enhances immune system and can help relieve migraines, asthma and sore muscles.

Coconut Sugar

Coconut sugar also know as Coconut Palm Sugar is made from the sap of cut flower buds of the coconut tree and has been used as a sweetener for thousands of years. Coconut sugar is subtly sweet with a hint of caramel but the taste varies depending on how it's processed. Coconut sugar contains magnesium, potassium, zinc, iron B vitamins, amino acids and is diabetic friendly.

The body processes all sweeteners the same so the benefit is in the taste and additional health benefits as opposed to one sweetener being healthier than another.

Become Successful On This Diet

Bloating is a constant problem especially for women. There are generally four causes for bloating: hormones, digestive conditions such as irritable bowl, colitis, etc., gas and believe it or not dehydration. Diuretics help to release water retained by the body and will help with temporary weight loss.

Hormonal bloating is part of women's monthly cycle and can be relieved by using herbs such as Black Cohosh and Donq Quai.

Bloating from digestive conditions can be countered by an herb called Cat's Claw or Una De Gato from Brazil. It's an anti-inflammatory that helps to calm irritated and inflamed digestive tracts and bowels to give relief from pain, gas, bloating and discomfort.

When you don't drink enough water your body thinks it's being dehydrated and will retain whatever fluid is in your body and will not let it go until it is convinced that it will not be deprived from water. So be sure to drink as much water as you can on this diet especially since coconut is a diuretic.

Diuretics

Green Tea

Green Tea is made from the unfermented leaves of the camellia flower. It comes in caffeinated and decaffeinated forms. Drink two or three cups a day or take supplement capsules which are naturally decaffeinated.

Dandelion Leaf

Dandelion is made from the same dandelions in your yard and is one of the most effective diuretics available. Dandelion contains essential vitamins and minerals including potassium, which is lost on commercial diuretics, and is free from any side effects. It comes in tea and capsules form.

Become Successful On This Diet

Stinging Nettle

Stinging Nettle is a plant and contains essential minerals including potassium, iron and magnesium. It's available in tea, capsule and tincture form which is an alcohol based herb extraction. In large quantities it can cause stomach upset.

Ginseng

Ginseng is not only used for cooking but is a natural appetite suppressant and Siberian ginseng works as a diuretic.

Thyme

Thyme is not only used for cooking but is a remedy for colds and flu in addition to being a great diuretic. It comes in capsule and powdered form.

Turmeric

Turmeric is a spice that's a good diuretic. It comes in capsule or powdered form for steeping as a tea.

Coffee

Both regular and decaffeinated coffee have zero calories and have diuretic properties due in part to the caffeine. Be sure to watch the sugar and creamer as that adds calories and can negate all your hard work.

Recipes

Here are some of my recipes. I am vegetarian but I have adapted them for both vegetarian and non-vegetarians. I am not a recipe follower as I season to taste, but I will list the basic recipes and I encourage you to experiment with these and other ingredients and spices to create your own version of these delicious recipes.

Vegetarian Salisbury Steaks with Brown Gravy

This is a strictly vegetarian recipe.

Preheat oven to 425

Vegetarian Burgers
2 tbls Flour
2 cups Water
1 tbls coconut or palm oil
2 cubes or 2 tsp. bouillon. I use Better Than Bouillon No Beef Base. It also comes in No Chicken Base base as well as Vegetable Base.
1 tsp Gravy Master or any brand browning and caramelizing seasoning
½ tsp salt
½ tsp pepper
½ tsp paprika
½ tsp rosemary
½ tsp thyme
½ tsp sage

Add flour and bouillon to water and mix to make a roux. Place in skillet and add oil and all your spices. Bring to a boil on medium heat stirring constantly. If gravy is too thick add more water by tablespoons full. If too thin add more flour by tablespoons full. Add salt and pepper to burgers, cover with gravy and place in oven for 15 minutes on each side.

Recipes

Oven Fried Chicken

Preheat oven to 425.

You can use either your favorite cuts of chicken or vegetarian chicken patties with this recipe. Oven frying uses less oil which means fewer calories. If there is a Seventh Day Adventist store in your area they have a mind boggling selection of meat substitutes in almost any form you can imagine. It's a wonderful resource for vegetarian food.

¼ cup palm or coconut oil
½ cup all-purpose unbleached flour
½ tsp salt
¼ tsp pepper
½ tsp rosemary
½ tsp sage
½ tsp thyme
¼ tsp paprika

Heat margarine in a rectangular or glass pan until melted. Mix flour and all spices in a paper or plastic bag. Place chicken in bag and shake to coat. If using pre-battered vegetarian chicken patties, forgo the flour and just sprinkle the spices over the patties. Place chicken in pan and bake uncovered 30 minutes on each side or until juices run clear. For vegetarian patties cook for 15 minutes on each side. For crunchier chicken, substitute cornflake crumbs for the flour and dip chicken in coconut or palm oil before shaking in the bag.

Recipes

Baked Fish

Preheat oven to 350 degrees.

1lb. Fish (fresh or frozen of our favorite type)
½ cup all purpose unbleached flour
3 tbls coconut or palm oil
½ tsp salt
¼ tsp pepper
¼ tsp garlic powder
¼ tsp paprika
¼ tsp sage
½ tsp lemon juice

Place oil in pan and place in oven to heat. Rinse fish and remove any remaining scales. Place flour and spices in a bag and place fish in bag and shake to coat. Place fish in pan or baking dish and bake for 20 minutes on each side until fish flakes with a fork, Sprinkle lemon juice on fillets if desired before serving.

Garlic Roasted Potatoes

Preheat oven to 450 degrees.

6 Potatoes washed and dried and cut in ¼ in strips
2 cloves thinly sliced garlic
2 tbls coconut or palm oil
½ tsp paprika
salt and pepper to taste

Peel potatoes and cut in fourths about 1 inch thick. Place in one layer in baking dish. Add garlic and oil and turn potatoes in oil making sure to coat each one. Sprinkle with salt, pepper and paprika. Bake for 30 minutes, turn potatoes over with a spatula and bake an additional 15 to 20 minutes or until tender and crispy.

Recipes

Farina Bread

This is a twist on Cornbread. It uses Farina or Cream of Wheat instead of cornmeal. Farina is easier to digest and makes a softer bread.

Heat oven to 350

1cup Farina
½ cup all purpose unbleached flour
1 ½ tbls baking powder
4 tbls sweetener
1 tsp salt
2 eggs beaten
3 tbls coconut or palm oil
1 tbls distilled white vinegar
1 cup plus 2 tbls buttermilk

Heat oil in a square or rectangle pan in your oven. Make buttermilk by adding 1 tbls distilled white vinegar to your milk. Stir and let sit for 5 minutes. Add dry ingredients in a large bowl and mix with a whisk to combine. Add eggs to buttermilk & if using honey add to buttermilk mixture. Pour buttermilk into dry ingredients and stir with a whisk to combine. Remove oil from oven and pour into the batter stirring quickly to combine without letting the oil cook the batter. Pour the batter back into your pan and bake for 30 minutes or until toothpick or fork stuck in middle come out clean. Cover Farina bread until ready to serve. This will help keep the bread soft and moist.

Recipes

Bran Muffins

Pre heat oven to 400 degrees.

1 1/3 cup all-purpose unbleached flour
½ cup sweetener or honey
1 tbls baking powder
1 tsp salt
1 ½ cup All Bran cereal
1 cup milk or milk substitute
1 egg
1/3 cup coconut or palm oil

Oil your baking pan with either coconut or palm oil. Pour bran and milk into a small bowl. Let sit for five minutes to soften bran. Add dry ingredients to a large bowl and mix with whisk to combine. Add egg to bran mixture along with honey if using instead of granulated sweetener. Stir to combine and add to dry ingredients. I like to use my hands. The mixture will be thick. If using muffin pans scoop about 1 tbls into each muffin opening. I prefer to pour the mixture into a large rectangular cake pan and spread out into pan like a sheet cake. Bake for 20 minutes or until toothpick or fork comes out clean. Remove muffins from pan or slice muffin sheet into squares, cover until ready to serve.

Recipes

Navy Bean Soup

1 lb navy beans
2 cans navy beans
1 large onion
4 carrots or 1 bag frozen carrots
1 green bell pepper
1 stalk of celery
¼ cup coconut or palm oil
1 4oz can tomato sauce
½ *tsp baking soda
1 bay leaf (optional)
1 tbls turmeric
1 tbls thyme
1 tbls curry
1 tbls ginger
1 tbls paprika
1 tbls cumin
1 tbls sage
1 tbls rosemary
1 package of Chili-O Mix
½ tsp black pepper
salt to taste

Wash beans and let stand in water overnight. Pour off water, place in Dutch Oven or pasta pot, cover with fresh water to top of pot, add baking soda and cook for 1 hour. Chop and sauté all vegetables in coconut or palm oil until onions are translucent and add all vegetables and spices to beans. Continue to cook for another hour or until beans and vegetables are tender.

*Baking soda removes gas from the beans. Use a spoon or ladle to scoop excess gas bubbles out of the pot and turn to medium high heat until the soup boils clear. Salting uncooked beans will cause them to be tough. This is a basic recipe. Please feel free to increase spice amounts as necessary to achieve desired flavor.

Recipes

No Bake Cheesecake

You can use either low-fat cream cheese or soy cream cheese (Tofutti) (shameless unpaid plug) to make this cheesecake.

1 8-9 inch pie pan
2 large glass or metal mixing bowls (chilled)

Graham Cracker Crust

1 ½ cup crushed graham crackers
2 tbls granulated sweetener (No Honey)
6 tbls palm oil

Cheesecake Filling

1 8 oz Soy Cream Cheese or Low-fat Cream Cheese
½ cup granulated sweetener
1 tsp pure vanilla extract
1 cup low-fat whipped cream, non-dairy whipped cream or coconut whipped cream (*see recipe below)

Crust

Grease bottom and side of a 8-9 inch baking pan with palm oil.

In a large bowl mix graham crackers, granulated sweetener and melted coconut/palm oil. Press graham mixture into bottom and sides of pan. Cover with plastic wrap and refrigerate.

Filling

Beat cream cheese with an electric mixer in a large chilled bowl until smooth. Add granulated sugar and beat till light and fluffy. Scrape sides of bowl and beat in vanilla. Fold in whipped cream. Pour filling into the chilled pie crust and smooth into crust. Cover and place in the refrigerator overnight to chill.

Recipes

*Coconut Whipped Cream

I've not had the opportunity to make this myself but I have a great recipe from a friend who has.

1 can Thai Kitchen Coconut Milk (Thai Kitchen is the only brand that is thick enough to freeze solid.)

½ to 2 cups powered coconut sugar (depending on sweetness) (place granulated coconut sugar in a blender or food processor and grind into powder)

½ to 1 tsp tsp pure vanilla extract

1 large glass or metal bowl chilled in freezer overnight

Do not shake can. Place coconut milk and a glass or metal bowl in the freezer overnight.

Open can (without shaking) and place coconut milk in chilled bowl. Add powdered coconut sugar and vanilla mix with electric mixer until light and fluffy. Fold into cream cheese mixture.

Summary

The Fabu Naturals Fat Burner Diet is a delicious and easy way to burn fat and lose weight. The shake is delicious and along with daily exercise, you are able to eat what you want (within reason) and lose weight. Once you've lost the weight, you can continue to drink the shake as a healthy addition to your daily diet. It's loaded with protein, potassium, calcium, probiotics, vitamins, minerals, calcium & iron to supplement even the busiest lifestyle.

Good Luck on your weight loss.

Please follow us on Twitter @fabunaturals and like on Facebook https://www.facebook.com/pages/Fabu-Naturals/434571833310304 for helpful articles on everything natural and herbal.

Bernique M. Johnson

Founder & CEO of Fabu Naturals